Intermittent Fasting
for Women over 50

A Guide to Intermittent Fasting and Increasing Your Metabolism and Energy Levels

Table of Contents

Introduction

Nutritionists used to recommend taking short, regular meals during the day and never miss them. Any of such experts have now changed their minds. They now advocate an alternative to diet scheduling known as intermittent fasting, or IF, which entails occasional brief fasts ranging from 14 to 48 hours and may provide significant health benefits.

Fad diets abound around the country. Diet pills were common in the 1990s. If you didn't get a juicer in your early twenties, you were losing out on life's critical wellness boosters. Green tea pads that minimize tummy size have been sent to us; even if you're not eating like a Neanderthal, you're still at a disadvantage. Intermittent fasting is a method of calorie restriction that involves a collection of on and off intervals of feeding. Although further research is needed, the early research on this eating pattern seems to be quite positive in terms of weight loss, but it might not be much more successful than merely reducing your daily calorie intake. For certain people, intermittent fasting is healthy, but it is not for all. Skipping meals of p regnant or breastfeeding females might not be the right way to lose weight. Consult the doctor until beginning intermittent fasting if you have gastroesophageal reflux, kidney stones, diabetes, or other medical issues.

It's an approachable fitness and weight-loss technique because it stresses meal schedules rather than avoidance of some ingredients. IF you boost your eating satisfaction in a variety of ways: With just the fasting timeframe to remember, you can notice that you are less concerned about what you consume in general.

Chapter 1: Intermittent Fasting And How It Works?

1.1 What Is Intermittent Fasting?

Intermittent fasting is a daily diet technique that alternates between fasting and eating. Research suggests that prolonged fasting is a way to control weight and avoid or even cure a certain type of disease. Most diets depend on whether to consume, but intermittent fasting is more about what you eat.

Through extended fasting, you just feed at a given period. Fasting for a set number of hours each day or eating just one meal a few times a week can help the body metabolize calories, and clinical evidence has shown that it can also provide health benefits. Mark Mattson, Ph.D.(Johns Hopkins)neuroscientist, has been intermittent fasting for 25 years.

He claims that our bodies have evolved to be able to go for many hours, days, or even weeks without eating. Before humans learned to evolve, they were hunter-gatherers who evolved to endure and prosper for long periods of time without food. Fifty years earlier, it was simpler to keep a healthier weight. People stopped feeding before going to bed, and there were no mobile and TV shows were turned off at 11 p.m. Portion sizes were much smaller. The bulk of citizens worked and played outside, and they usually had more activity."

TV, phone, and other sources of content are also available 24 hours a day, seven days a week. We sit up late watching videos, playing sports, and talking on the phone. We enjoy the whole day and half of the night lying and snacking."

Increased risk of type 2 diabetes, obesity, heart disease, and other ailments may be linked to consuming more calories and doing less. Intermittent fasting has been shown in studies to further reduce these patterns.

1.2 What Is the Process of Intermittent Fasting?

Intermittent fasting may be done in a variety of ways, but they both depend on selecting regular feeding and fasting periods. For instance, you might consider feeding the only period every day and fasting the remainder. You could even limit yourself to one meal a day over an eight hour, 2 times a week. Intermittent fasting can be done in a variety of ways.

According to Mattson, the body reduces its sugar stores and starts to burn fat during hours without food. This was alluded to as metabolic tossing by him.

"For several other Americans, who feed during their daytime hours, intermittent fasting corresponds to the daily dietary plan," Mattson says. "If somebody eats three meals a day, plus desserts, but does not work out, they are running on all of those calories and not losing weight."

Intermittent fasting functions by extending the period until the body has absorbed all of the calories consumed during the previous meal and has begun to burn fat.

When we feed, more nutritional energy is ingested than will immediately be utilized. Any of this energy must be put up for later use. Insulin is the main hormone associated with the storage of food energy.

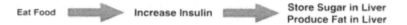

Insulin increases as we feed, helping to contain the extra energy in two different forms into glucose (sugar) units that can be linked together to form long chains to form glycogen, which is then stored in the muscle or liver. There is, though, very little storage capacity for carbohydrates, and if it is reached, the excess glucose is transformed into fat by the liver. De-novo Lipogenesis is the name given to this mechanism. (meaning simply "making new fat").

Any of this freshly produced fat is retained in the liver, but much of it is transported to other fat storage in the body. Despite the fact that this is a rather complicated process, it seems there is no limit on the number of fat which can be produced. So, two important food energy storage mechanisms operate in our bodies. One is readily available but with minimal storage space (glycogen), while the other is more difficult to reach but has nearly limitless storage space (body fat).

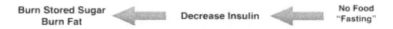

The mechanism goes in reverse when we do not feed. Insulin levels decrease, signaling the body to start burning accumulated energy when no more is coming from food. Blood glucose sinks because the body must now take glucose out of storage to burn for energy. Glycogen is the most readily available energy source. It is broken down into glucose molecules to supply nutrition for the body's other cells. This will supply enough energy to fuel most of the body's needs for 24 to 36 hours. After that, the body would mainly be breaking down fat for energy.

So the body resides in two systems - the fed condition and the fasted state. Either we are accumulating food storage (increasing stores) or burning stored energy (decreasing stores). It's one or the other. If feeding and fasting are balanced, so there should be no net weight gain. If we start feeding the minute we roll out of bed and do not pause until we go to sleep, we spend nearly all our time in the fed state. Over time, we may accumulate weight because we have not given our body any time to burn stored food fat.

To regain equilibrium or reduce weight, we can raise the average time spent burning food energy. That's intermittent fasting. In fact, intermittent fasting encourages the body to utilize surplus fat. The main point to consider is that there is nothing problematic with that. That is how our bodies are made. That's what dogs, cats, lions and bears do. That's what people do.

If you're eating every third hour, which is always advised, your body can continuously utilize the incoming food resources. It does not need to burn much body fat, if any. You might only be accumulating fat. Your body could be storing it for a period when there is little to eat. If this occurs, you neglect equilibrium. You neglect intermittent fasting.

1.3 Intermittent Fasting Can Help Weight Loss

To achieve the weight reduction goals, the majority of people want intermittent fasting. IF is an excellent way of losing weight easily and improve your health. How is it going to work? It's just quite easy. You begin by consuming fewer calories by following a fasting diet plan, which lowers your overall daily calorie intake. This drastic change in your lifestyle causes important changes in your body, which help you lose weight.

The body tends to use refined body fat for fuel instead of sugars from carbohydrates while you're fasting. IF aims to optimize insulin synthesis in this way. According to the report, hormonal changes allow short-term fasting to raise metabolism from 3.6 to 14%. The lower level of insulin makes stored body fat quite accessible. Fasting helps to lower insulin levels. This reduces fat retention and allows the body to utilize stored fat. As a consequence, keeping a low and healthy insulin level is important for weight loss. You would be able to lose weight so quickly comfortably.

IF makes common sense, the food we consume is broken down by enzymes in our stomach which ultimately winds up as molecules in our bloodstream. Carbohydrates, especially sugars and refined grains (think white flour and rice), are easily broken down into sugar that our cells use for energy. If our cells don't need it all, they preserve it in our fat cells. Sugar will only reach our cells with insulin, a hormone produced in the pancreas. Insulin takes fructose into the fat cells and retains it there.

During meals, as long as we don't eat, our insulin levels can go down, and our fat cells will then release their accumulated sugar for use as energy. We lose some weight if we let our sugar level goes down. IF's whole idea is to encourage the insulin levels to go down high enough and for long enough that we burn off our weight.

1.4 Why Intermittent Fasting Is Good For Your Body?

There are also advantages involved with fasting for weight reduction. But you'd be mistaken to believe this is the only explanation that intermittent fasting is appropriate for you. Here you will read more about legitimate explanations why you need it.

It's Easier than Dieting

Maybe you've done everything you can to stick to a diet, but nothing seems to work. It's not always easy to stick to a diet that involves reducing portion sizes, so losing weight or being better isn't always about calories. It's more important to change what you eat than how many times you feed. Intermittent fasting is easy if you understand how to do it.

Besides that, it is convenient to create a dieting timetable, but it is challenging to adhere to it. You might have a hard time locating the food you like at particular hours, or you may be lacking in excitement. An intermittent type fasting program, on the other hand, seems to be a big roadblock. It is, nevertheless, quick to achieve. For one instance, a diet typically involves eliminating 'harmful' ingredients and eating fewer carbohydrates. Doesn't it appear to be quick? But what happens when the hunger pangs strike? Consuming even more than you like at defined intervals is a convenient and healthy alternative. Nonetheless, try to eat in balance and excess calories can just slow down the weight loss process.

Fasting Intermittently Is Less Stressful

Imagine beginning the day thinking you've got a lot to plan before breakfast. That's the routine of dieting, which may eat up a large portion of the day. Fasting, on the other side, is easy, transparent, and less exhausting. On other days, fasting means consuming one fewer meal. So, you're free of any stress to cook at particular times throughout the day.

It May Reduce Adverse Health Condition Risks

Obesity is among the critical causes in various forms of harmful health problems. Intermittent fasting, though, assists with weight loss and insulin regulation. Therefore, by reducing more body weight, people can reduce the chance of heart attacks and diabetes. Besides, other effects include reduced blood pressure and improved cholesterol levels. It is important to remember, though, that intermittent fasting may not be appropriate for people with such health issues. As a result, before beginning a fasting regimen, speak with your doctor about how safe and beneficial this could be to you.

1.5 How to Implement Intermittent Fasting?

After focusing your mind on fasting, it's time to execute the routine. Health is the overall focus, so make sure you do the following before continuing your intermittent fasting diet.

Choose Easy Options

It is essential, particularly if it's your first time. Depending on what you're fine with, you can keep it easy. This even goes for meals. It's not a rigid diet, but you can consume much of your daily meals. However, make sure you get adequate nutrients and fluids and restrict diets rich in sugar, saturated fats, salt, cholesterol etc. For starters, consuming diet soda is doubted a smart idea, while keeping hydrated is crucial. Of course, you want the right mix of meals to help you have the perfect out of your fast.

Your reason for fasting is also important and making things simpler to obey. For starters, your motivations for fasting may involve weight reduction, to prevent some illnesses, including heart conditions, or to survive better.

See an Expert or a Doctor

Your health is at risk here. Rather than rush into a fasting regimen, discover what's best for the body. This way, you can realize what you can manage. For starters, if you have a medical problem like diabetes, get a professional opinion. Besides, whether you're under treatment or sound ill through the procedure, try quitting.

Figure Out the Days And Times

It would be best if you focused on the periods you eat on your calendar. This way, there are no mishaps. More so, pick moments you're familiar with. For instance, you may enjoy eating your first meal at 1 pm when your second meal falls in at 8 pm.

The days of the week even matter. Most specialists vote for weekdays. Maybe it's because the days are packed with tasks, so you won't have time to interrupt the schedule or worry about health. This sounds fine, but you should follow other days to meet your needs. For starters, you can make do with time-restricted eating.

1.6 The Science Behind It

Studies suggest that intermittent fasting can be a very effective weight-loss technique. A 2014 analysis study showed that this eating behavior would induce 3 to 8 percent weight loss over 3 to 24 weeks. According to the same report, people have lost 4–7 percent of their waist circumference.

It is said that studies investigating fasting are calling for more human studies, particularly large-scale human studies. Many of the purported effects of intermittent fasting come from laboratory trials or small-scale animal studies, which have not been confirmed in broader cohorts. In comparison, while weight reduction appears like the most promising upside, some claims are debatable.

For instance, decades of research on rodents have shown that intermittent fasting can help them stay lean, acquire less aging-related diseases, and live 30-40 percent longer. A 2019 analysis of studies in the New England Journal of Medicine found that intermittent fasting would lower blood pressure and cholesterol levels, enhance mental function, decrease inflammation, and increase stamina. But experiments on people have been less definitive. It appears to be ideal for dropping excess pounds, but everything else is less obvious.

However, and so, bear in mind that the biggest explanation for its popularity is that intermittent fasting makes you consume fewer calories overall. If you drink and consume excessive quantities through your feeding hours, you can not lose much weight at all.

1.7 Intermittent Fasting Provides Anti-Aging Benefits

Researchers found that reducing calories increased energy output and reduced the risk of chronic diseases, such as cardiac failure, diabetes, and cancer when performing experiments on the effects of calorie reduction in overweight adults. Probing further, they discovered that limiting calories reduced cellular harm and helped preserve stable DNA. These are two main factors in combating aging since weakened and inflamed cells contribute to chronic disease, whereas aging begins as DNA wears down.

While calorie restriction can provide anti-aging benefits, remaining on a diet that includes lowering your caloric consumption by 30 to 40 percent and keeping with this every day for the long run isn't possible for most people. In the quest for an alternative to calorie restriction, intermittent fasting soon appeared as a choice. It provides the same life-extending advantages without placing unreasonable nutritional demands.

1.8 The Impact Of Intermittent Fasting On Your Body

Beneficial modifications arise at the molecular level while the body is fasting, even though the fast is brief or sporadic. The following shifts, which are caused by intermittent fasting, function together to encourage a healthy and long life:

Gene expression: Changes occur in genes that promote longevity and prevent disease.

Cellular repair: Cells remove more wastes that would cause cellular damage.

Protects against oxidative stress: Prevents cell damage due to unstable molecules called free radicals.

Fights inflammation: Intermittent fasting decreases inflammation.

Hormonal changes: Drop-in insulin levels prevent diabetes and may boost longevity.

Intermittent fasting frequently lets you shed weight and belly fat, which in turn increases your fitness and eliminates chronic ailments that can prolong your existence.

1.9 Anti-Aging Benefits Of Calorie Restriction

CR (calorie restriction) is the most powerful of all anti-aging treatments.

Traditional CR, as we discussed in how to fast and what to expect during intermittent fasting, reduces calories by 20-40% for extended periods of time, which is neither recommended nor normal among bio hackers due to mental divergence.

Many previously unknown pathways of aging have been revealed in humans and animals as a consequence of the CR report. According to a well-written and systematic report in Clinical Interventions of Aging titled Will eating less help you live longer and better? Calorie restriction encourages five main mechanisms affecting healthy aging. Calorie limitation has been updated:

- Inflammation: NF-kb
- Antioxidants: Nrf2

- Mitochondrial physiology: AMPK / SIRT
- Cell Proliferation: IGF-1 and TOR (specifically mtor)

- Autophagy: foxo
- It's worth noting that all of these mechanisms are interrelated.

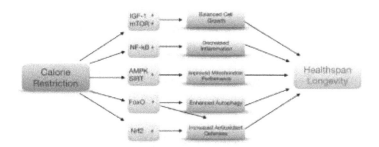

Studies also found that the most significant part about fasting is the cellular advantages that you reap from offering the body a rest. Galvin says this begins with the cell's mitochondria, the portion of the cells that turn food into energy. These have their DNA which can get exhausted when we consume too much, but fasting gives them a chance to regenerate, which delays aging on a cellular basis. According to one critical piece of research, too much body fat may even overtake the mitochondria and speed up aging. At the same time, fasting has the opposite impact.

So no matter what you consume, fasting will help the cells regenerate and heal, the study showed. But to reduce weight, Galvin says that the only approach to make the most of your fasting is to maintain your blood sugar stabilized and your food balanced. "So if someone is eating too many high carb foods and not enough fat or protein, you can have a blood sugar spike," she says, which signals the body to accumulate fat, undoing all the better intentions.

1.10 Intermittent Fasting Lets Cells Repair, Helps Avoid Disease

If you intermittent fast, you are literally allowing your body and your cells a chance to heal from stress and toxins. Your cells' mitochondria get to heal, which leads to healthy cells and disease control," Galvin explains. "And letting the body repair itself is very great for brain health as well," she adds. Studies have shown that fasting will reduce the lab's age-related cognitive decline, although these studies have been on mice so far. As for the aging process, fasting has caused excitement since DNA gets damaged in two ways: by genetics and through behavior. The behavioral kind of what's helped through fasting.

In the cells, mitochondria help turn the food we consume into energy, so when it gets weakened, it's vulnerable to mutations, according to recent studies. "Because mitochondrial DNA has a limited ability to repair itself when it is damaged, these mutations tend to build up over time," according to a report reported in Genetics Home Research, part of MedlinePlus.

"A buildup of somatic mutations in mitochondrial DNA has been correlated with certain types of cancer and an elevated risk of some age-related diseases such as cardiac disease, Alzheimer's disease, and Parkinson's," the study found. "Additionally, evidence indicates that the gradual accumulation of these mutations over a person's lifespan may play a role in the natural phase of aging. According to the findings, helping your body to fast is a way to reduce the risk of cancer and slow down the aging process.

Chapter 2: Intermittent Fasting - Types And Benefit

2.1 Types of Intermittent Fasting

The very first element you can consider is a meal schedule that you are more comfortable with. Nutritionists established many different types of intermittent fasting feeding routines as a result of its popularity. Most of them seem to be effective. However, you must decide which one is the perfect match for you.

2.1.1 Intermittent Daily Fasting
14:10

For women, this approach is supposed to be the most powerful. You can feed at 10 a.m. and fast from 8 p.m. to 10 a.m. the next day. If you can't survive without breakfast, though, this strategy isn't for you.

THE 14:10 DIET

	DAY 1	DAY 2	DAY 3	DAY 4	DAY 5	DAY 6	DAY 7
MIDNIGHT 4 AM	FAST	FAST	FAST	FAST	FAST	FAST	FAST
10 AM 12 PM	First meal	First meal	First meal	First meal	First meal	First meal	First meal
4 PM	Last meal by 8PM	Last meal by 8PM	Last meal by 8PM	Last meal by 8PM	Last meal by 8PM	Last meal by 8PM	Last meal by 8PM
8 PM MIDNIGHT	FAST	FAST	FAST	FAST	FAST	FAST	FAST

16:8

Men get the strongest outcomes following this 16:8 solution. You should consume anything you like within an 8-hour feeding window and fast for the remaining 16 hours. Typically, a fasting time coincides with the evening meal at about 8 P.M. before noon the following day. It would be best if you changed your eating routine; for example, you might consume all the meals between the time span of 11 AM and 7 PM. An often raised query is, "How often should I do the 16:8 fasting?" It is a daily fasting diet plan, so you are supposed to do it every day to see weight loss results. Remember, intermittent fasting is not a diet; it's an eating routine that can become a part of the lifestyle.

THE 16/8 METHOD

	DAY 1	DAY 2	DAY 3	DAY 4	DAY 5	DAY 6	DAY 7
Midnight / 4 AM / 8 AM	FAST	FAST	FAST	FAST	FAST	FAST	FAST
12 PM	First meal	First meal	First meal	First meal	First meal	First meal	First meal
4 PM	Last meal by 8pm	Last meal by 8pm	Last meal by 8pm	Last meal by 8pm	Last meal by 8pm	Last meal by 8pm	Last meal by 8pm
8 PM / Midnight	FAST	FAST	FAST	FAST	FAST	FAST	FAST

20:4

This procedure requires 4 hours of feeding and 20 hours of fasting. For starters, you will have your meals around 2:00 pm and 6:00 pm every day and fast for the remaining 20 hours. This way, you will have one or two simple meals in your 4-hour feeding gap.

2.1.2 Alternate Day Intermittent Fasting

This approach requires longer fasting times. Typically, people go for 24 to 36 hours without calories, only one meal a day. However, the biggest drawback to this strategy is that it's very difficult to obtain all the necessary nutrients from one meal. A well-balanced diet includes a lot of cooking. Moreover, it's very difficult to get enough calories with only one single meal a day, so a 24-hour cycle of fasting is quite hard for a dieter.

ALTERNATE-DAY FASTING

DAY 1	DAY 2	DAY 3	DAY 4	DAY 5	DAY 6	DAY 7
Eats normally	24-hour fast OR Eat only a few hundred calories	Eats normally	24-hour fast OR Eat only a few hundred calories	Eats normally	24-hour fast OR Eat only a few hundred calories	Eats normally

2.1.3 Weekly Intermittent Fasting

If you are new to intermittent fasting, then this approach would be the simplest one for you. This technique is not as successful as frequent intermittent fasting; however, you can still get loads of benefits from it. The concept is very easy. Typically, people adhere to this method quickly for 24 hours and consume just once a day. This approach can be used 2-3 times a week. For starters, you may start the fasting period at pm on Friday and get your first meal at noon on Sunday. Consequently, you miss about 2-3 meals per week but beware that this approach won't help you lose weight.

2.1.4 Eat-Stop-Eat
5:2

This diet strategy's core premise is that you have five daily eating days and two fasting days. You will consume up to 500 calories a day at any point during the fasting days. What to eat on fasting days? Make sure the diet is well-balanced to contain protein, salad, fruits, and high-fiber items. Don't always try to fast two days in a row as it won't be successful; try to split them.

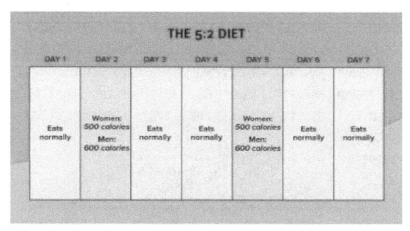

2.1.5 Spontaneous meal skipping

You don't need to pursue a formal intermittent fasting regimen to enjoy any of the rewards. Another choice is to miss meals from time to time, such as when you don't feel hungry or are too distracted to prepare and eat.

It's a fallacy that people ought to feed every few hours lest they enter hunger mode or lose muscle. Your body is well able to endure long stretches of starvation, let alone to miss one or two meals from time to time. Thus, if you're just not hungry one day, miss breakfast and only have a good lunch and dinner. Or, if you're traveling anywhere and can't locate something you want to consume, do a small fast. Skipping one or two meals when you feel tempted to do so is simply a random intermittent fast.

SPONTANEOUS MEAL SKIPPING

	DAY 1	DAY 2	DAY 3	DAY 4	DAY 5	DAY 6	DAY 7
	Breakfast	Skipped Meal	Breakfast	Breakfast	Breakfast	Breakfast	Breakfast
	Lunch	Lunch	Lunch	Lunch	Lunch	Lunch	Lunch
	Dinner	Dinner	Dinner	Dinner	Skipped Meal	Dinner	Dinner

2.1.6 The Warrior Diet

Ori Hofmekler, a fitness expert, made popular the Warrior Diet . It involves consuming limited amounts of fresh vegetables and fruits during the day and one main meal at night. In turn, you fast during the day and feed at night within a four-hour eating window. Among the first conventional diets to include extended fasting was the Warrior Diet. The dietary habits of this lifestyle are similar to that of the paleo diet, with a focus on the whole, unprocessed foods.

THE WARRIOR DIET

	DAY 1	DAY 2	DAY 3	DAY 4	DAY 5	DAY 6	DAY 7
Midnight / 4 AM / 8 AM / 12 PM	Eating only small amounts of vegetables and fruits	Eating only small amounts of vegetables and fruits	Eating only small amounts of vegetables and fruits	Eating only small amounts of vegetables and fruits	Eating only small amounts of vegetables and fruits	Eating only small amounts of vegetables and fruits	Eating only small amounts of vegetables and fruits
4 PM	Large meal	Large meal	Large meal	Large meal	Large meal	Large meal	Large meal
8 PM / Midnight							

2.1.7 Overnight Fasting

As the name indicates, you will fast for 12 hours. This period normally comes at nighttime, while you sleep, which allows it the most convenient means of fasting to implement. It's also named autophagy fasting because of the 12-hour time cycle, which primarily benefits the cells. A great benefit of this form of fasting is that it's quick to start. Besides, it's good for lowering calorie consumption, as well as for weight reduction.

2.2 Best Foods To Eat While Intermittent Fasting

First, let's take a step back to break down the basics: How does the diet function when it comes to these big intermittent fasting health benefits? Scientists postulate that the anti-aging effects are primarily attributed to improved insulin regulation, and weight reduction is linked to an overall decreased calorie consumption because of a shorter feeding window. Simply placed, because you have less time throughout the day to prepare, you eat less. But a central concept, as in any diet, is assessing viability for your lifestyle. There are several best foods to build the ultimate intermittent fasting diet guide to avoid nutritional shortfalls.

1. Water

One of the most critical facets of sustaining a balanced eating habit during intermittent fasting is to encourage hydration. As we go without energy for 12 to 16 hours, our body's preferred energy supply is the sugar accumulated in the liver, also known as glycogen. If this energy is burned, so disappears a huge amount of fluid and electrolytes. Drinking at least eight cups of water a day can reduce dehydration and also encourage improved blood flow, memory, and muscle and joint strength during your intermittent fasting regimen.

2. Lentils

This healthy superstar delivers high fiber power with 32 percent of total regular fiber needs fulfilled in just half a cup. Besides that, lentils provide a good source of iron (about 15 percent of your daily needs), another nutrient of concern, particularly for active females experiencing intermittent fasting.

3. Minimally-Processed Grains

Carbohydrates are an important aspect of life and are most likely not the threat when it comes to weight loss. Since a big chunk of your day would be spent fasting during this diet, it's crucial to think carefully about how to get enough calories while not getting too complete. While a balanced

diet minimizes refined foods, there will be a time and place for things like whole-grain bread, crackers, and bagels and since these foods are more easily digested for fast and simple fuel. If you plan to exercise or workout frequently during intermittent fasting, this can particularly be a good source of energy on the go.

4. Hummus

One of the softest and best-tasting snacks known to mankind, hummus is another outstanding plant-based protein and is a perfect way to increase the nutrient value of classics like sandwiches; just swap it in for mayonnaise. If you're brave enough to create your hummus, don't ignore that the trick to the best recipe is tahini and garlic.

5. Potatoes

Comparable to bread, white potatoes are metabolized with minimum effort from the body. And if combined with a protein source, they are a great post-workout snack to refresh starving muscles. Another advantage that makes potatoes an important choice for the IF diet is that once cool, potatoes shape a resistant starch prepared to feed beneficial bacteria in your gut.

6. Smoothies

If a daily supplement doesn't sound enticing, consider springing for a double dose of vitamins by preparing organic smoothies filled with fruits and vegetables. Smoothies are a perfect way to ingest several different foods, each individually filled with different essential nutrients.

7. Blueberries

Never let their miniature appearance confuse you: Blueberries are evidence that good stuff comes in small packages! Studies have found that survival and youthfulness were a function of anti-oxidative mechanisms. Blueberries are a perfect source of antioxidants, and wild blueberries are also one of the best sources of natural antioxidants. Antioxidants help detox the body of free radicals and avoid widespread cellular harm.

8. Vitamin D Fortified Milk

The recommended consumption of calcium for an adult is 1,000 milligrams a day, exactly what you'd receive from consuming three cups of milk per day. With a shortened eating window, the chances to consume this much may be rare, and so it is necessary to choose high-calcium foods. Vitamin D fortified milk increases the body's processing of calcium which can help to keep bones healthy. To increase regular calcium consumption, you can add milk to desserts or cereal or just

consume it with meals. If you're not a fan of the drinks, non-dairy options rich in calcium include tofu and soy goods, as well as leafy greens like kale.

9. Ghee

You've known a drizzle of olive oil has huge health benefits, but there are lots of other oil varieties out there you can use, though. You don't want to heat the oil you're cooking with above its smoke point, so next time you're in the kitchen heating up a stir-fry, try using ghee as your oil of preference. Basically, all clarified butter; has a far higher smoke point making it a better substitute for hot dishes.

10. Papaya

You may encounter hunger symptoms in the last hours of your fast, particularly if you're just starting out with intermittent fasting. This "hanger" will potentially contribute to major overeating, making you tired and irritable minutes away. Papaya produces a particular enzyme called papain, which acts to break down proteins. Incorporating parts of this tropical fruit into a protein-rich meal will aid absorption and reduce bloating.

11. Branch Chain Amino Acid Supplement

The BCAA is a final IF approved substitute. While this muscle-building aid is best for athletes who enjoy fasted cardio or vigorous workouts first thing in the morning, it may be consumed at any time during the day (fasting or not) to prevent catabolism and preserve lean muscle mass. Notice that this product might be off-limits if you choose to pursue a vegan diet since much of it is produced of duck feathers.

2.3 Intermittent Fasting Plan

Here is the Intermittent Fasting Plan that offers you action for each day with a thorough explanation to support you kick-off your Intermittent Fasting journey in a simple, enjoyable and sensible manner.

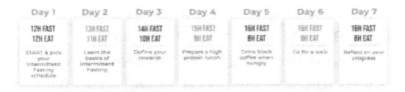

Day 1	Day 2	Day 3	Day 4	Day 5	Day 6	Day 7
12H FAST 12H EAT	13H FAST 11H EAT	14H FAST 10H EAT	15H FAST 9H EAT	16H FAST 8H EAT	16H FAST 8H EAT	16H FAST 8H EAT
START & pick your Intermittent Fasting schedule	Learn the basics of Intermittent Fasting	Define your rewards	Prepare a high protein lunch	Drink black coffee when hungry	Go for a walk	Reflect on your progress

DAY 1

TODAY'S TASK: 12 h Fast | 12 h Eat

TODAY'S MISSION: Pick your Intermittent Fasting schedule

You can progressively incorporate intermittent fasting throughout the first week. This is why we suggest starting with a 12 hour fast on the first day and eventually rising to 16 hours on Day 5 by introducing one hour every day. It is safer for the body and brain to become accustomed to various diet plans this way; additionally, you grant yourself more time to become accustomed to Intermittent Fasting.

We also would like you to select an Intermittent Fasting plan that ideally matches your lifestyle and that you will commit to for the entire 21 days Intermittent Fasting Journey from the first day.

Consistency has proved to be one of the most contributing factors of progress.

DAY 2

TODAY'S TASK: 13 h Fast | 11 h Eat

TODAY'S MISSION: Learn the basics of Intermittent Fasting

Your swift will be extended to 13 hours on Day 2. You should do it in only one hour more than you did yesterday! Day 2 is a great day to get you into some healthy eating habits that can help you achieve your Intermittent Fasting objectives: just focus on consuming more whole foods and avoiding the usual suspects, including fat, processed foods, and hollow carbohydrates.

We can give you a collection of typical meals and foods you should consume to get improved Intermittent Fasting outcomes. Think basic but delicious and nutritious meals you can make at home, such as poached eggs with spinach, meatballs with zucchini noodles, feta cheese salad or homemade hummus for a snack.

DAY 3

TODAY'S TASK: 14 h Fast | 10 h Eat

TODAY'S MISSION: Define your rewards

Rewards are important when developing a current Intermittent Fasting habit. Hence on Day 3, we were hoping you could determine your own reward for each effectively fasted day.

Why are rewards so important?

A reward sends a constructive signal to the brain, saying, "Doing this feels good. We should do more of it!" It might be something that makes you feel nice.

Ideally, the right Intermittent Fasting benefit can be linked to the primal needs for relaxation, socializing, food or playing.

The reward may also be quick (but powerful!) The celebratory gesture you do soon after finishing the habit, including cheering yourself up and saying "Good job" or checking just another day off of your regular success monitoring sheet you get after joining the task.

If the reward is smaller, for example, dinner at an expensive but so tasty restaurant, you might pursue a token strategy, e.g., every good day fasting "gives you" 1 token. When you have earned five tokens, you get to reward yourself and head out to the restaurant.

DAY 4

TODAY'S TASK: 15 h Fast | 9 h Eat

TODAY'S MISSION: Prepare a high protein lunch

You'll have also fasted for 15 hours on Day 4 of Intermittent Fasting! To break your hard, eat a high-protein snack that will help you meet your weight loss goals. You may make sauteed or grilled veggies with a protein of your choices, such as meat, fish, legumes, beans, eggs, tofu, almonds, grilled beef, and seeds, for example. If you're looking for some recipes, how about this refreshing summer pomegranate salad with wild salmon?

DAY 5

TODAY'S TASK: 16 h Fast | 8 h Eat

TODAY'S MISSION: Drink black coffee when hungry

On Day 5 of the intermittent fasting Plan, you'll eventually hit the overall 16/8 intermittent schedule of fasting for 16 hours and feeding for 8 hours. And it will be relatively simple to do, as we have seen in ourselves and hundreds of those who have completed the 21-Day Intermittent Fasting Task.

If you're having trouble getting through the 16-hour quick and quenching your hunger, we recommend consuming black coffee. It's high in antioxidants which will help you lose weight (but don't overdo it!).

Keep in mind the coffee for Intermittent Fasting is dark. This means no sugar, syrup, or creamers, no cappuccino, latte, or flat white, only black coffee. If you must have something tasty, use the organic sweetener stevia, but be cautious because it can trigger hunger.

Are you a non-coffee drinker? Choose a cup of green or black tea or a glass of water.

DAY 6

TODAY'S TASK: 16 h Fast | 8 h Eat

TODAY'S MISSION: Go for a walk

Are you hoping to lose weight through these 21 days of fasting? It is important to eat a well-balanced diet, and we recommend that you have some exercise in your daily routine. Just before you break your fast, go for a stroll. Even a brief 20-minute walk will suffice. Walking is an excellent way to improve your physical fitness, improve your mood, and actually have some fresh air. Most importantly, going for a walk will distract you from your appetite and make the last few hours of fasting go more smoothly.

DAY 7

TODAY'S TASK: 16 h Fast | 8 h Eat

TODAY'S MISSION: Go for a walk

Maintain the latest 16/8 IF plan today, and by doing so, concentrate on your week's gains. Taking a full-body picture, logging your weight, and comparing them to the initial weight and image are both parts of the accomplishment process. You can begin to see the first signs of weight loss and/or a change in your physical appearance. In addition, we'd like you to address a few questions regarding your success, such as how you're doing, whether intermittent fasting has changed your stamina, attitude, or skin, and so on.

Going through an exercise like that would help you recognize when, and most significantly, why you might be struggling and, therefore, help you take steps to accelerate your results and make intermittent fasting a new sustainable habit.

2.4 What To Eat For Breakfast?

When you're about to break your fast, it's better to ease out of it. To stop overloading the digestive tract, incorporate small quantities of more easily digested foods at the end of your fast. Break your fast with foods that are heavy in calories, sugar, or perhaps even fiber may be tough for your body to digest, triggering bloating and discomfort. Foods and beverages that may be much more surprising to the system after a fast include those like a stinky cheeseburger, piece of cake, or soda. Also, high-fiber fresh food, nuts, and seeds can be challenging to digest.

Nutrient-dense foods that are simple to absorb and have a small amount of protein and good fats, on the other side, will help you break the fast more easily.

Below are a few examples of what to eat to break your fast.

Smoothies. Blended drinks can be a gentler way to introduce nutrients to your body since they contain less fiber than whole, raw fruits and vegetables.

Soups. Soups that contain protein and easily digestible carbs, such as lentils, tofu, or pasta, can gently break a fast. Avoid soups made with heavy cream or a large amount of high-fiber, raw vegetables.

Dried fruits. Dates are a concentrated source of nutrients frequently used for breakfasts in Saudi Arabia. Apricots and raisins may have similar effects (21Trusted Source).

Fermented foods. Try unsweetened yogurt or kefir.

Breaking your fast with healthy foods that may be better tolerated can help replenish important nutrients and electrolytes while easing food back into your diet.

Healthy fats. Foods like eggs or avocados can be great first foods to eat after Vegetables. Cooked, soft, starchy vegetables like potatoes can be good food options when breaking a fast.

Chapter 3: Pros And Cons Of Intermittent Fasting

There are several various types of IF, ranging from systems where food is entirely omitted on certain days to procedures where food is only limited during certain periods of the day. The different lifestyle habits have gained recognition to achieve and sustain a stable weight and reap fitness benefits even among already balanced individuals.

3.1 Pros

3.1.1 Easy to Follow

Often dietary preferences depend on consuming specific items and restricting or excluding other foods. Learning the basic rules of an eating style will entail a considerable time investment. For example, there are whole books dedicated to understanding the DASH diet or discovering how to execute a Mediterranean-style meal schedule. In a diet schedule that involves extended fasting, you actually feed according to the time of day or day of the week. If you've decided which intermittent fasting method is better for you, all you need is a watch or a calendar to know what to feed.

3.1.2 No Macronutrient Limitations

There are common eating plans that dramatically limit particular macronutrients. For example, many people adopt a low-carb diet plan to improve fitness or lose weight. Others practice a low-fat diet for health or weight loss purposes. Each of these plans allows the user to follow a different style of eating, sometimes changing preferred items with new and potentially unknown foods. This could entail new cooking learning skills to shop and store the kitchen differently.

Neither of these skills is needed when intermittent fasting solely because there is no targeted macronutrient level, and no macronutrient is limited or prohibited.

3.1.3 Could Potentially Boost Longevity

One of the most commonly cited effects of intermittent fasting includes durability. According to the National Institute on Aging, rodent experiments have shown that when mice are placed on programs that heavily limit calories (often during fasting periods), several show an extension of lifespan and reduced rates of many diseases, particularly cancers.

So does this advantage apply to humans? According to those who promote the diets, it does. However, long-term research is required to validate the advantage. According to a study published in 2010, there has been empirical evidence connecting religious fasting to long-term longevity effects, but it was hard to ascertain whether fasting offered the boost or whether similar factors played a role.

3.1.4 No Calorie Counting

Not unexpectedly, individuals who are attempting to achieve or sustain a healthier weight normally tend to stop calorie counting. Although nutrition labels are readily found on many items, the task of calculating portion sizes and tabulating regular counts either manually or on a mobile app may be tedious.

Research published in 2011 showed that people are more inclined to adopt plans when all pre-measured calorie-controlled meals are delivered. Commercial diets such as WW, Jenny Craig, and others offer these programs for a price. But often, families don't have the money to pay for these types of services, particularly long term.

Intermittent fasting offers a convenient option where little to no calorie-counting is needed. In certain cases, calorie restriction (and consequently weight loss) arises when food is either removed or greatly reduced on certain days or at certain hours of the day.

3.1.5 Promotes Weight Loss

In a study of intermittent fasting research published in 2018, investigators note that the findings they studied demonstrated a substantial decrease in fat mass among participants who engaged in clinical trials. They also noticed that intermittent fasting was found to be effective in lowering weight, independent of the body mass index. The study also stated that while short-term weight reduction was checked, longer-term trials are required.

Intermittent fasting could be no more successful than other diets that limit calories daily. A 2018 research contrasted intermittent fasting with conventional diets (defined as constant energy restriction) and concluded that weight loss benefits are comparable.

In a major meta-analysis conducted in 2018, scientists analyzed the findings from 11 trials lasting between 8 to 24 weeks. Study authors found that both intermittent fasting and constant energy restriction obtained similar outcomes if weight loss and metabolic changes were the targets. They suggested that longer-term studies are required to draw conclusive conclusions.

It is also likely that weight-loss outcomes can rely on age. Research reported in the journal of Nutrition in 2018 investigated the impact of intermittent fasting (time-restricted feeding) on

young 20-year-old and older 50-year-old males. Intermittent fasting marginally reduced body mass in the youth, but not in the older men. However, muscle strength remained the same in both classes.

3.1.6 Unrestricted Eating

Anyone who has ever modified their diet to obtain a medical gain to hit a healthier weight understands when you tend to desire things that you are advised not to consume. In reality, a report published in 2017 concluded that an intensified drive to diet is a major contributor to failed weight loss attempts. But this challenge is strictly constrained on an intermittent fasting schedule. Food deprivation only applies during such limited hours, and on the nonfasting hours or days of the plan, you will usually consume anything you want. In reality, researchers also name these days feasting days.

Of course, consuming fatty things would not be the healthiest way to reap advantages from intermittent fasting, but taking them out on those days restricts the total diet and may ultimately benefit.

3.1.7 Glucose Control

In 2018, several intermittent fasting studies claimed that this eating pattern may help people with type 2 diabetes control blood sugar by weight reduction in overweight or obese persons but may exacerbate insulin sensitivity in healthy people.

A case series released in 2018 showed the efficacy of fasting (accompanied by medical monitoring and 6-hour long dietary training) to reverse insulin resistance while retaining regulation of their blood sugars over a seven-month cycle. In all three scenarios, patients were able to end insulin treatment, lose weight, lower belly size, and see an overall increase in blood glucose.

However, another report conducted in 2019 found a less remarkable effect on blood glucose regulation with greater sample size and with continuous medical advisement. Researchers performed a 24-month follow-up to a 12-month experiment contrasting extended fasting with prolonged calorie reduction in people with type two diabetes. They observed that hba1c levels grew in both the constant calorie restriction and sporadic groups at 24 months.

These observations were compatible with evidence from other research indicating that it is not unusual for blood glucose levels to rise over time in people with type 2 diabetes through a variety of nutritional treatments. However, the study authors do notice that intermittent energy restraint might be superior to continuous energy restriction for retaining lower hba1c levels but noted that further research with larger sample sizes is required to validate the advantage.

3.1.8 Other Health Benefits

Some findings have linked intermittent fasting with a number of other health benefits. However, almost all study author notes that further analysis is required to properly appreciate the value. For example, one research reported in 2018 reported that intermittent fasting during Ramadan contributed to the reduction of total LDL, triglycerides, cholesterol in study subjects. The participants have gained an improvement in HDL levels.

Another 2014 study showed that intermittent fasting (specifically time-restricted feeding) could be an efficient approach to tackle low-grade systemic inflammation and certain age-related chronic diseases linked to immune function without losing physical performance. Notice that this has only been tested in 40 men, and a wider version analysis remains to be performed.

3.2 Cons

Studies exploring the implications of intermittent fasting often refer to some adverse effects that may arise during the fasting stage of the feeding routine. For example, it is not unusual to feel moody, heartburn, suffer nausea, sleepy, constipation, dehydration, decreased sleep quality, or anemia. If you have asthma, elevated LDL cholesterol levels, an abnormally high amount of uric acid in the blood, cardiovascular disease, hyperglycemia, and liver and kidney disorders, intermittent fasting may be harmful.

3.2.1 Reduced Physical Activity

One important consequence of intermittent fasting could be the lack of physical exercise. Most intermittent fasting systems do not provide a requirement for physical exercise. Not unexpectedly, those who adopt the plans may feel such exhaustion that they struggle to achieve everyday step targets and may even adjust their normal workout habits.

A continuing study has been suggested to *see* how intermittent fasting can influence physical activity habits.

3.2.2 Medications

Many patients who take medicines feel that taking a medicine with food tends to alleviate those side effects. In reality, certain prescriptions clearly bear the suggestion that they should be consumed with food. Therefore, taking medicines during fasting can be a problem.

Anyone who takes medication should talk to their healthcare professional before beginning an IF procedure to ensure that the fasting stage would not interact with the medication's efficacy or side effects.

3.2.3 Severe Hunger

Not unexpectedly, it is normal for those in the fasting phase of an IF eating routine to feel extreme hunger. This hunger can become more intense when they are around those who are eating normal snacks and meals.

3.2.4 May Promote Overeating

During the "feasting" stage of many intermittent fasting methods, meal size and meal duration are not limited. Instead, customers indulge in an ad libitum diet. Unfortunately, this can encourage overeating in some individuals. For example, if you feel hungry after a day of full fasting, you may feel tempted to overeat (or eat the wrong foods) on days when "feasting" is required.

3.2.5 No Focus on Nutritious Eating

The key to any intermittent fasting strategies is pacing instead of food choice. Therefore no foods (including those that fail good nutrition) are avoided, and foods that offer good nutrition are not encouraged. For this cause, those adopting the plan don't actually learn to consume a balanced diet.

Suppose you are pursuing a short-term intermittent fasting regimen for weight reduction or to achieve a medicinal advantage. In that case, it is not possible that you can practice specific healthy eating and cooking skills, like how to cook with healthy oils, how to consume more veggies, and how to select whole grains over processed grains.

3.2.6 Long-term Limitations

While the practice of intermittent fasting is not new, much of the research investigating the eating style's advantages are only recently discovered. As a result, it's difficult to say if the gains would last. Additionally, researchers often comment that long-term studies are needed to determine if the eating plan is even safe for more than several months.

For now, the safest course of action is to work with your healthcare provider when choosing and starting an IF program. Your medical staff will keep track of your results and any health advantages or problems you might have to make sure that the eating style is healthy for you.

3.3. Common Intermittent Fasting Myths

If you're doing intermittent fasting or contemplating doing it, it's vital to get the right detail. With the truth in mind, you're more able to fast properly. And when you fast correctly, you're more likely to enjoy the weight loss, stable energy, and decreased cravings that have made intermittent fasting common. Unfortunately, there's plenty of misinformation out there. You've already read stuff like: Fasting delays your metabolism, you should not drink water on a fast or, fasting shrivels up your muscles.

These fasting theories, though, aren't rooted in fact. Instead, they're focused on rumor, conjecture, and a misguided emphasis on traditional wisdom.

Myth #1: fasting decreases your metabolism

Some people fear that fasting reduces the resting metabolic rate (in other terms, that fasting helps you burn fewer calories at rest) (in other words, that fasting makes you burn fewer calories at rest). The fear is that you'll put on weight like a three-toed sloth when you start regularly eating again. This is what occurs on calorie restriction diets, which means consuming 50 to 85 percent of the calories the body consumes on a long-term regular basis. Your body adapts to the reduced energy consumption, and it will remain that way for years.

If you've ever watched The Biggest Loser, you've seen calorie reduction in reality. The contestants lose weight, but they nearly always win it back. Inconveniently for fans, they never discuss the aspect of the program.

Does the same happen for intermittent fasting? It appears not. In a 2005 report conducted in the American Journal of Clinical Nutrition, non-obese people who observed alternate-day fasting retained a regular metabolic rate for the majority of three weeks, even while burning more fat.

Myth #2: you shouldn't drink water while fasting

Some religious fasts, including Ramadan fasting, require both food and water restriction. Perhaps unrelated, a host of arguments have surfaced that no-water fasts are optimal for wellbeing.

Unfortunately, because fasting has a diuretic impact, restricting water may contribute to dangerous dehydration. That's why doctors pay particular attention to fluid consumption when supervising patients undertaking clinical fasts. Physicians often pay particular attention to electrolytes like sodium and potassium, all of which are energetically peed out during fasting.

. Drink water during a run, and try supplementing potassium and sodium fasts longer than 13 or 14 hours.

Myth #3: you can't gain muscle while fasting

Fasting doesn't feel like the right way to develop muscle. After all, don't you continue to pound protein shakes? Ok, you definitely need nutrition, so you don't need it 24/7. In one 2019 report, for instance, healthy people following 16/8 fasting gained almost as much muscle and power as women feeding on a more traditional schedule. Here's the issue. Your body works intensely to conserve muscle in periods of shortages. When you are hard, you switch to body fat (not muscle) for energy needs. Think of it this way: If humans burnt out muscle during a fast, our ancestors might have been too frail to hunt!

Myth #4: fasting makes you overindulge

After a fast, you'll be hungry. This appetite, many think, would fuel future overeating. The data, however, doesn't support this concern. Most fasting studies encourage patients to consume as much as they want a procedure called ad libitum eating. They eat their fill, and they still lose weight. In reality, you'll actually consume less, not more, on most intermittent fasting protocols. This moderate calorie restriction, in particular, encourages gentle weight reduction without slowing the metabolism.

Myth #5: it's for everyone

Intermittent fasting is common right now. In certain ways, it's being sold as good for all countries, all the time. But though fasting is safe and nutritious for most individuals, some groups should stay clear. These classes include:

- Children
- Pregnant and nursing women
- Underweight people

The above groups need to consume more food, not less. The chance of nutritional loss outweighs any possible fasting advantages. Many of those who have elevated blood sugar can still continue with caution. Though fasting may be therapeutic for this community, medical care is necessary to avoid dangerously low blood sugar (hypoglycemia) from arising.

Myth #6: fasting *saps* your energy

Food is fuel. Without it, won't the energy levels plummet?

Eventually, indeed. But as you fast intermittently, the cells tap into an alternative energy source: body fat. And there's plenty of it to go around. That's correct. And a slim individual (e.g., 150 pounds with 10 percent body fat) has amazing fat reserves to meet energy requirements when fasting. If you do the calculations, 15 pounds of fat corresponds to over 60,000 calories of energy!

In reality, many people report good energy when they workout in a fasted state. It makes sense, given that blood is drawn away from tissues and into digestive organs during a big meal.

Myth #7: you can't focus while fasting

Look back to that time you were ferociously starving. It really wasn't the most zen moment. But if you follow a daily practice of extended fasting, you shouldn't feel this "hungry" condition. When your cells transition to utilizing body fat for nutrition, your appetite hormones stabilize.

Burning body fat often releases ketones, small molecules that fuel the brain with pure, usable energy. Promoting a condition of ketosis, it's been shown, increases concentration, memory, and emphasis in older adults.

Myth #8: Don't shower or wash your hair during confinement

New mums are also advised not to wash their hair or even shower while in isolation, out of the misconception that doing so would enable 'wind' to penetrate the body and inflict joint or bone pain. If you're a soon-to-be mother, you would be happy to learn that this is just an ancient wives' story without factual justification.

Bathing provides good sanitation and decreases the likelihood of skin and wound diseases, which may not result in joint discomfort of any sort. If you are ever cautious, just ensure that you do not bathe in water that is too cold instead of skipping baths or showers entirely.

Myth #9: Eggs contribute to high cholesterol

Eggs have received an undeserved poor rap. There is inadequate evidence to prove that dietary cholesterol intake (such as that in eggs) influences our blood cholesterol levels. Our unhealthy cholesterol levels are more affected by the intake of saturated and trans fat. It is essential to hold your cholesterol in balance by controlling these fats in your diet.

On the other side, eggs are an economical source of several nutrients, including omega-3 fatty acids, copper, iron, antioxidants and vitamin D. Nevertheless, eggs contain saturated fat and should be consumed in moderation; a balanced individual can consume up to 6 eggs per week, as a reference.

Myth 10: Eating spicy food can give you stomach ulcers

It is no doubt that many want their food spicy, so this is actually positive news for many contrary to common belief; spicy food is not one of the triggers of stomach ulcers. Stomach ulcers are normally the product of infections attributable to the Helicobacter pylori (H. Pylori) bacteria, not spicy food. Other variables like family background, obesity and excessive drinking may affect the chances of developing ulcers. It is necessary to remember, however, even if you still have an ulcer, it is also better to avoid spicy food.

Chapter 4: Intermittent Fasting And Working Out

Exercise has its own fitness benefits; it's normal why you might want to keep a daily workout schedule when fasting.

4.1 Things to Know About Intermittent Fasting and to work Out

Here are eight things you should know about safely and effectively working out while fasting.

1. Continue working out while fasting. But take it easy

Fasted exercises have their advantages. Working out on an empty stomach may help with weight loss because your body would depend on stored food in the form of glycogen and fat instead of burning your most recent meal. When exercising in a fasted state, though, there is a risk your body will start breaking down muscle for food. That's because high-intensity exercises depend on carbohydrates for power. That means running sprints or doing your daily Crossfit exercise during fasting or at the end of your fast can reduce your workout's benefits. You can even be less energized to work out intensely if you're new to IF.

So though fasted high-intensity weight lifting can have negative effects, low-intensity cardio works mainly on fat. The perfect intermittent fasting exercises for cardio include biking, jogging, meditation, swimming and gentle Pilates.

2. Listen to your body

If you have some health conditions (especially those that can trigger dizziness, including low blood sugar or low blood pressure), work out when fasting would not be in the cards. Pay attention to your body, and do what feels good! If you do feel weak during exercise out, rest, refill, and hydrate before initiating IF or before bringing in the workout to the IF schedule, check with your doctor or healthcare professional to advise what's best for you.

3. Start adapting to a fat-burning metabolism

Suppose you like to combine keto and IF; stop starting all at the same time. It takes a couple of weeks for your body ro respond to any adjustments or new habits, so adopt low-carb living before fasting to allow your body time to adapt. If you experience some chronic fatigue, weakness, dizziness, depression, burnout, bruises, nausea, or are slow to heal from your workouts, it's time to pull it down a level. Intermittent fasting and exercise can be daunting to handle. And be warned: extra workouts can leave you feeling hungrier in general, which can make fasting much more challenging, particularly if the intensity is too strong.

4. Hydration

It is essential to drink lots of water and electrolytes while fasting, particularly while fasting and working out. Headaches, low blood sugar, nausea, dizziness, low blood pressure, and cramping may occur if the electrolytes aren't controlled properly. Replenish electrolytes with organic coconut water, electrolyte capsules, or zero-calorie electrolyte beverages. Avoid sports beverages that are rich in calories as well as caffeine and other diuretics. Make sure you are eating enough sodium and potassium along with being properly hydrated.

5. Refuel on protein after a workout

Improve your fast by consuming enough protein, high fiber carbohydrates, and balanced fats during your fueling windows. Follow up your higher intensity exercise with protein within 30 minutes of completing the workout. If you're performing moderate-intensity cardio with an empty stomach, work out at the close of the fasting time so you can refuel straight after. Keep to a whole, organic foods that balance protein and carbohydrates. We like scrambled eggs with vegetables, or if you are on the go and in need of a fast and easy post-workout fueling solution, consider a protein bar or protein shake.

6. Time of day you prefer to work out

If you're someone who just works out pre-8 a.m., you may need to change your feeding hours so you can enjoy a meal right after an aerobic exercise. If you're a lover of afternoon workouts, that's a sweet place for weight lifting. Low-intensity exercises should be completed at every time of day.

7. Vary your workouts

It's helpful for the body to do a combination of strength training and exercise to gain muscle while still blasting fat. This will support you on your IF plan, too. For days where you can get in a morning exercise, concentrate on cardio, and on days when you need to visit the gym in the evening, physical exercise is your BFF. When you're feeling extra depleted, miss your exercise or try meditation or Pilates instead.

8. Use electrolytes

Low-calorie choices like coconut water or natural sports beverages will help make sure your body is getting electrolyte refueling without breaking your fast.

4.2. How To Pick The Right Workout For The IF Plan

Not all exercise is the same when it comes to scheduling it with the intermittent fasting method. Some forms of workout appear to be more depleting for the muscles, and these may include a meal immediately afterward or a higher carbohydrate consumption earlier in the day.

Cardio and HIIT

When performed right, fasted cardio can be a perfect addition to the fitness routine. And depending on which sort of exercise you perform, you can or may not require a meal immediately afterward. If you're off for a slow and steady morning run, you could be OK waiting many hours after your exercise to start feeding. But if that makes you feel weak and dizzy, consider eating a meal right after you stop working out. Like every hard exercise on this new diet, it's necessary to *ease* into it. "If people have a tonne of hypoglycemia when they don't feel well while they've fasted, easing into fasted cardio will take some time. You have to prepare the body to be able to reach these fasted conditions.

Yoga, barre, and low-intensity workouts

On days where you're feeling lower in energy, even throughout the time when you're first transitioning to intermittent fasting, low-intensity exercises may be better on the body, either in a fasted condition or during your eating window. If you're searching for a quick exercise to blend in across the fasted window of the day, these can be fantastic choices. Those seem to be much more fasted [than weight training]. People who tend to practice intermittent fasting maybe a couple of days a week perform even better because they do things like barre, Pilates, meditation, and they can hold it in their fasting window, versus needing to also be able to replenish nutrition and protein in strength-based exercises or high intensity based workouts.

Strength training

In order to build muscle mass, it's necessary to boost your metabolism with protein and refined carbs, either before working out or immediately afterward. "If someone is working to improve mass and stamina, then they ought to do the exercise either just before they break their fast or in their diet plan, not towards the close of their eating window where they then can't heal from that. Doing your strength training through your feeding window will mean your muscles have enough power to perform the job without breaking down.

It just boils down to what helps you feel best. You have to balance; what are your fitness goals? How do you like to feel during your workout, and how do you really feel during your workout?" If you realize that you're completely exhausted, and therefore you can't successfully work out, something's not correct. Having a little bit of food before could serve you to really meet those weightlifting goals or the HIIT exercise target you have. In this scenario, afternoon or evening exercises would suit well with your schedule.

4.3. Schedule To Get The Most From Fasting And Working Out

Monday: cardio followed by a protein-rich breakfast

Tuesday: lunch with complex carbs, p.m. Strength training followed by dinner

Wednesday: yoga, barre, Pilates, or other low-intensity workouts

Thursday: cardio followed by a protein-rich breakfast

Friday: lunch with complex carbs, p.m. Strength training followed by dinner

Saturday or Sunday: yoga, barre, Pilates, or other low-intensity workouts

This schedule depends on your specific fasting needs and can be adjusted according to what works best for you.

4.4. Intermittent Fasting Mistakes

1. Starting off drastically with intermittent fasting

Starting out dramatically is one of the greatest errors you can create. If you rush into IF without *ease* into it, you can set yourself up for catastrophe. Going from consuming three regular-sized meals or 6 smaller meals a day to eat within a four-hour span, for example, could be a difficult change.

Instead, *ease* into fasting steadily. If you are going for the 16/8 process, progressively extend the hours between meals so you can easily fit within a

12-hour timeframe. Then, to reduce the time to 8 hours, add few minutes every day before you get to the 8 hour cycle.

2. Not choosing the right plan for intermittent fasting

You're able to pursue Intermittent Fasting for weight reduction and have supermarket shopped for entire grains like fish and poultry, fruits and vegetables, and nutritious sides like quinoa and legumes. The thing is, you haven't selected the IF strategy that will put you up for success. If you are a committed gym-goer, six days a week, absolutely fasting for two of those days might not be the perfect plan.

Rather than leap into a plan without thought, evaluate your lifestyle a little and choose the plan that would suit your routine and behavior better.

3. Eating too much in your fasting window

One of the reasons why people want to try Intermittent Fasting would be that the cost and time left to eat means consuming few calories. However, a few other people will eat their regular amount of calories throughout the span of the fasting window. This may mean that you'll never lose some weight.

Don't consume your regular consumption of 2000 calories in the window. Conversely, intend to eat around 1200 to 1500 calories during the time frame when have breakfast. However, many meals you eat would then depend on the fasting window's length, whether that be 4, 6, or 8 hours. If you really need to overeat and are in a condition of deprivation, rethink the schedule you decide to follow, or *ease* off the IF for a day to refocus, then get back on track.

4. Eating the wrong foods in your fasting window

Overeating goes hand in hand with the Intermittent Fasting missteps of eating the wrong foods. You will not feel well if you have a fasted state window of 6 hours and fill it with balanced, fatty, or sugary foods. The cornerstone of your diet becomes lean proteins, healthy fats, nuts, legumes, unrefined grains, and wholesome vegetables and fruits. In addition, when you're not fasting, keep these healthy eating tips in mind:

- Avoid processed foods and cook whole foods instead
- Read nutrition labels and become familiar with forbidden ingredients like high fructose corn syrup and modified palm oil
- Cook and eat at home as opposed to in a restaurant

- Balance your plate with fiber, healthy carbs and fats, and lean proteins
- Watch your sodium intake and beware of hidden sugars

5. Restricting calories in your fasting window

There is such a phenomenon as calorie restriction that is unnecessary. It's not safe to eat fewer than 1200 calories during your fasting window. Not just that, but it has the potential to slow down your metabolic rate. If you delay your metabolism so long, you'll start losing muscle mass instead of gaining it.

6. Unknowingly breaking the intermittent fast

It's essential to be conscious of hidden fast breakers. Did you realize that even the flavor of sugar makes the brain release insulin? This triggers the release of insulin, essentially breaking the high. Here are some unexpected foods, supplements, and items that can stop a fast and trigger an insulin response:

- Vitamins, such as gummy bear vitamins, contain sugar and fat
- Using toothpaste and mouthwash containing the sweetener xylitol
- Supplements that contain additives like maltodextrin and pectin
- Pain relievers such as Advil can have sugar in the coating.

Breaking the fast is a common Intermittent Fasting error. When you're not feeding, clean your teeth with a baking soda and water mixture and closely scan the labels before consuming vitamins and supplements.

7. Not drinking enough when intermittent fasting

IF requires that you stay hydrated. Keep in mind that the body isn't absorbing the water that will normally be absorbed with food. As a result, if you're not patient, side effects might throw you off. If you cause yourself to become dehydrated, you can experience headaches, muscle cramps, and extreme hunger. Include the following in the day to prevent this error to avoid unpleasant signs, including cramping and headaches:

- Water
- Water and 1-2 tbsp of apple cider vinegar (this may even curb your hunger)
- Black coffee

- Black, herbal, oolong, or green tea

8. Not exercising when intermittent fasting

Some people believe they can't exercise during an IF time, when in fact, it's the perfect situation. Exercising makes you burn fat that has been accumulated in your body. Additionally, when you exercise, the Human Growth Hormone levels rise, assisting in muscle growth. There are, though, certain guidelines to obey in order to get the most out of the workouts.

To get the best results from your efforts, keep these points in mind:

- If the type of exercise is intense, make sure you eat before to make your glycogen stores available.
- Base your exercise on the fasting method; if you are doing a 24 hour fast, do not plan an intensive activity that day.
- Time your workouts for during the eating periods and then eat healthy carbs and proteins within 30 minutes of the exercise.
- Listen to your body's signals; if you feel weak or light-headed, take a break or conclude the workout.
- Stay hydrated during the fast and especially during the workout.

9. Being too hard on yourself if you slip when intermittent fasting

One snafu does not imply loss! You'll have days where an IF diet is especially difficult, and you don't think you'll be able to keep up. It's perfectly acceptable to take a rest if necessary. Set aside a day to start focusing. Stick to the balanced food plan, but indulge in surprises like an amazing protein smoothie or a plate of healthy steak and broccoli the next day.

Don't fall into the trap of having Intermittent Fasting take over your whole life. Consider it a component of your good routine; just don't forget to take care of yourself in other ways. Enjoy a good read, get some exercise, spend more time with your mates, and live as healthily as possible. It's just part of the process of being the strongest version of yourself.

Chapter 5: Delicious Recipes

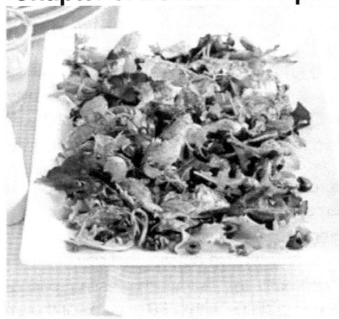

5.1. Potato And Paprika Tortilla

Cooking time: 25 minutes

Servings: 4

Difficulty level: Easy

Ingredients

- 6 large eggs
- 3 tbsp olive oil
- 250g new potato, thickly sliced ends trimmed
- 2 chopped garlic cloves
- 1 small halved and sliced onion
- ½ tsp of smoked paprika
- ½ tsp of dried oregano (or 3 tbsp of chopped parsley
- Few extra leaves for garnishing (optional)

Steps

1. In a deep 20centimetres non-stick frying pan, heat the oil. Cook the potatoes, onion, and garlic in a skillet for 10 minutes or until tender. Stir in paprika and cook for another minute.

2. Season the eggs with the dried or some fresh herbs, then pour them into the pan. When the

   the egg begins to set on the pan's bottom, stir about a couple of times, then cover and cook gently over a

3. very low flame for 10 minutes, or until set, other than the top.
4. Place the tortilla on a plate with care. Transfer to the pan and an uncooked top on the surface, and cook for another 1-2 minutes. Cover in foil.
5. Serve warm or cool while garnished with parsley if desired.

5.2 Lemony Mushroom Pilaf

Cooking time: 30 minutes

Servings: 4

Difficulty level: Easy

Ingredients

- 1 lemon juice and zest
- 1 sliced onion
- 2 garlic cloves
- 200g mixed rice (basmati) & wild rice
- 300g sliced mixed mushrooms
- 500ml vegetable stock
- 6 tbsp of light soft cheese also with garlic & herbs
- Small bunch of snipped chives

Steps

1. In a non-stick pan, heat 2 teaspoons of the stock, fry the onions for 5 minutes or soften.
2. If it begins to dry out, add a splash of stock. Cook for another 2 minutes after adding the mushrooms and garlic.
3. Mix in the rice, as well as the lemon zest and juice. Bring the remaining stock, along with the seasonings, to a boil.
4. Reduce heat to low, cover, and cook for 25-30 minutes, or until rice is soft.

5. Half of the chives and soft cheese must be stirred in, then serve with the unused chives and soft cheese on top.

5.3. Spiced Carrot And Lentil Soup

Cooking time: 15 minutes

Servings: 4

Difficulty level: Easy

Ingredients

- 125ml milk (fat-free)
- 140g red lentils (split)
- 2 tbsp of olive oil
- 2 tsp of cumin seeds
- 600g carrots (coarsely grated but no need to peel)
- Hot vegetable stock (cube)
- Pinch chili flakes
- Plain yogurt & naan bread for serving

Steps

5   Dry-fry 2 tsp of cumin seeds as well as a pinch of the chili flakes in a big saucepan for 1 minute, or before they start to hop around and unleash their aromas.

6   Using a spoon, scoop out about half of the mixture and put it aside. Bring 2 tsp olive oil, 600 grams thinly sliced grated carrots, 140 grams split red lentils, 1-liter hot vegetable stock, and 125 milliliters milk to a boil in a saucepan.

7   Cook for 15 minutes, or until the lentils are softened and darkened.

8   Using a stick blender or a food processor, puree the soup until creamy (or if you prefer, leave it chunky).

9   Season to taste, then top with a dollop of yogurt as well as a sprinkling of the toasted spices that were set aside. Hot naan or bread is a great accompaniment.

5.4   Pineapple With Thai Prawns And Green Beans

Cooking time: 15 minutes

Servings: 2

Difficulty level: Easy

Ingredients

- 1 tbsp of vegetable oil
- 100g pineapple chunks (fresh)
- 100g of green bean
- 100g of whole cherry tomato
- 2 lemongrass stalks (remove the tough outer leaves and rest are finely chopped)
- 200g of raw king prawn
- A small pack of Thai basil leaves (or regular basil leaves)
- A thumb-sized piece of ginger (shredded)

For the sauce

- 2 tbsp liquid chicken stock
- 1 tbsp of fish sauce
- 1 tbsp of soft brown sugar
- tbsp of lime juice (wedges to serve)

5.5   Paillard Chicken With Lemon And Herbs

Cooking time: 20 minutes

Servings: 6

Difficulty level: Easy

Ingredients
-
- 1⁄2 tbsp of balsamic vinegar
- 140g of bag rocket
- 2 tbsp of olive oil
- 25g parmesan
- chicken breasts (skinless)
  Lemon wedges

For the marinade
-
- 2 garlic cloves
  3 rosemary sprigs (finely chopped leaves)

- sage leaves (finely shredded)
- 1 lemon juice & zest
- 3 tbsp of olive oil

Steps

6. Every chicken breast should be sandwiched between two sheets of cling film or baking parchment. Flatten each chicken piece with a meat mallet or rolling pin to an even layer about 0.5cm thick. Place in a serving bowl.
7. To create the marinade, use a pestle and mortar to grind the garlic with a pinch of salt. Add the rosemary and sage and pound all together. Combine the lemon juice, olive oil, and freshly ground black pepper in a mixing cup. Pour the marinade over the chicken to make sure it's fully covered. Refrigerate for at least 2 hours after coating.
8. Preheat the barbecue. Add coals. Cook for 1-2 minutes on either side of the chicken. Shift to a board and set aside for a few minutes to cool.
9. In a big mixing cup, combine the oil and balsamic vinegar. Season with salt and pepper and add the rocket. Mix all together, then shave the Parmesan on top. Serve the salad with chicken and lemon wedges for squeezing.

5.6   Broccoli And Green Kale Soup

Cooking time: 20 minutes

Servings: 2

Difficulty level: Easy

Ingredients

-
- ½ tsp ground coriander
- 1 lime (zested & juiced)
- 1 tbsp of sunflower oil
- 100g kale (chopped)
- 2 garlic cloves (sliced)
- 200g courgettes (roughly sliced)
- 3cm piece of turmeric root - grated
  1/2 teaspoon ground turmeric

- 500ml stock (formed by mixing 1 tbsp of bouillon powder & jug of boiled water)
- 85g broccoli
- Pinch of a pink Himalayan salt
- Small roughly chopped pack parsley (but reserve the few whole leaves for serving)
- A thumb-sized piece of ginger (sliced)

Steps

5   In a deep skillet, heat the oil and add ginger, garlic, turmeric, coriander, and salt. Cook for 2 minutes on medium heat, then add 3 tablespoons of water to moisten the spices.

6   Stir in the courgettes, make sure they are properly coated in all of the ingredients, then cook for another 3 minutes. Simmer for 3 minutes after adding 400ml stock.

7   Pour the remaining stock over the kale, broccoli, and lime juice. Cook for another 3 to 4 minutes, or until all of the vegetables are tender.

8   Remove the pan from the heat and stir in the chopped parsley. Blend everything in a high-powered blender until smooth. Lime zest & parsley are optional for garnishing.

5.7   Spiced Chicken And Pineapple Salad

Cooking time: 10 minutes

Servings: 2

Difficulty level: Easy

Ingredients

-
- 1 red chili (deseeded & chopped)
- 1 small red onion (halved & thinly sliced)
- 1 tbsp of sweet chili sauce
- 2 tbsp of white wine vinegar
- 227g-can of pineapple juice
- 90g bag of mixed leaf
- 140g pack of cooked & sliced chicken breast
- Handful cherry tomatoes (halved)
  Small bunch coriander (leaves picked)

Steps

6. Drain the pineapple juice and set it aside. Chop the rings into pieces if they're in rings. If serving as a snack, mix the chicken, onion, leaves, coriander, and tomatoes in a mixing bowl

and split into two containers.

7. To make the dressing, mix 2 tsp pineapple juice, red chili, vinegar, and sweet chili sauce in a shallow jam jar or lidded bottle with some seasoning, and before serving, toss with the salad.

5.8   Acquacotta

Cooking time: 40 minutes

Servings: 4-6

Difficulty level: Easy

Ingredients

-
- 1 red onion (finely chopped)
- 2 garlic cloves (finely chopped)
- 2 small carrots (chopped)
- 2 tbsp parsley (chopped)
- 2 tsp thyme leaves (plus extra to serve)
- 225g plum tomatoes (deseeded & chopped)
- 3 celery sticks (chopped)
- 3 slices of crusty bread, toasted & torn into chunks
- 3 tbsp of olive oil
- 50g of dried porcini mushrooms
- 6 eggs
  850ml chicken stock

Steps

5   In a big saucepan, heat the olive oil and gently cook the celery, onion, garlic, carrots and thyme for bout 10-15 minutes, or until it becomes softened. Meanwhile, soak the porcini for 15 minutes in hot water until softened & swollen. Drain the mushrooms and finely cut them, reserving the soaking juice. Cook for another 5 minutes with the softened vegetables and the soaking liquid.

6   Add the tomatoes, then cook for 10 minutes, or before they start to break

down, and add the stock, then bring to a slow boil.

7   In another large saucepan, poach the 6 eggs for 3-4 minutes, or until set, now remove with the slotted spoon. Toss in the parsley and a pinch of salt and pepper, as well as torn-up the toasted bread. Distribute the soup among 6 bowls and top each with an egg. Serve with a sprinkling of fresh thyme.

5.9   Teriyaki Salmon Parcels

Cooking time: 20 minutes

Servings: 4

Difficulty level: Easy

Ingredients

-
  - 2 tbsp of low-salt soy sauce
  - 1 tbsp of clear honey
  - 1 garlic clove (finely chopped)
  - A little sunflower oil
  - 300g of Tenderstem broccoli
  - 4 ×100g of salmon fillets
  - 1 small ginger piece (cut into matchsticks)
  - Sliced spring onions (toasted sesame seeds)
    Cooked rice (for serving)

Optional:

-
  - A little sesame oil
    1 tbsp mirin

Steps

1. Prepare the marinade and sauce. Set aside a little bowl containing the soy sauce, butter, garlic, and mirin.
2. Cut some foil squares out. Cut 4 squares of aluminum foil, each about 30centimetres square, with scissors. Brush a little oil onto each sheet of foil to pull the edges up a little.
3. Fill the parcels to the maximum. Place a few broccoli stems on top of each one, then a salmon fillet and ginger on top.
4. Pour the sauce on top. Pour the sauce on each salmon fillet and, if

desired, drizzle with

sesame oil.

5. Close the packs. To seal the parcels, fold the foil edges together and position them on a baking sheet. It's possible to schedule it up to a day ahead of time.
6. Prepare the parcels. Preheat oven to 200°C
7. Let cook the parcels for 15-20 minutes, then removes them and leaves them to cool for a few minutes. Place each packet on the plate and open it. Serve with rice on the side and a sprinkle of spring onions & sesame seeds.

5.10. Ricotta, Tomato And Spinach Frittata

Cooking time: 35 minutes

Servings: 4

Difficulty level: Easy

Ingredients

- 1 tablespoon of olive oil
- 1 large onion (sliced)
- 300 g of cherry tomatoes
- 100g of spinach leaves
- A small handful of basil leaves
- 100 g ricotta
- 6 eggs beaten
- Salad (for serving)

Steps

5   Preheat oven to 200°C or 180°C.

6   In a big non-stick frying pan, heat the oil and fry the onion for about 5-6 minutes, or until tender and golden. To soften the tomatoes, put them in for 1 minute.

7   Turn off the heat and put the spinach leaves, then basil to wilt a bit. In an oiled 30cm × 20cm rectangular baking tin, mix all of the ingredients. Dot the ricotta over the vegetables in little scoops.

8   Season the eggs and whisk them thoroughly before pouring them over

the vegetables & cheese. Cook for 20 to 25 minutes in the oven or until lightly golden. Serve with a salad.

5.11. Sea Bass With Chili Sizzled Ginger & Spring Onions

Cooking time: 30 minutes

Servings: 6

Difficulty level: Easy

Ingredients

- 6 sea bass fillets (140g/5oz each with skin & scaled)
- 3 tbsp of sunflower oil
- Large ginger knob (peeled & shredded in matchsticks)
- 3 garlic cloves (thinly sliced)
- 3 fresh red chilies (deseeded & thinly shredded)
- Bunch spring onion (shredded long-ways)
- 1 tbsp of soy sauce

Steps

5   Salt and pepper 6 sea bass fillets, then slash a skin three times.

6   Heat 1 tbsp of sunflower oil in a heavy-bottomed frying pan.

7   When the oil is heated, fry the sea bass fillets while keeping the skin-side down for 5 minutes, or when the skin is crisp & golden. The fish will be almost completely fried.

8   Flip & cook for a further 30 seconds to 1 minute before transferring to a serving plate to stay warm. The sea bass fillets can be fried in two batches.

9   In a big skillet, heat 2 tsp of sunflower oil, and fry the big knob of peeled ginger, 3 garlic cloves (thinly sliced) and 3 red chilies (thinly shredded) for about 2 mins or until golden, then cut into matchsticks,

10   Remove the pan from the heat and add the shredded spring onions.

11   Put 1 tbsp of soy sauce on the fish and spoon on the pan's contents.

5.12. Squash Salad & Beetroot With Horseradish Cream

Cooking time: 45 minutes

Servings: 12

Difficulty level: Medium

Ingredients

- 6 red onions
- 50ml of olive oil
- 2 tbsp of red wine vinegar
- 1kg raw Beetroot
- 1-¼kg large butternut squash (peeled & deseeded)
- 1 tbsp of soft brown sugar

For the horseradish cream

- 1 lemon juice
- 175ml of soured cream
- 3 tbsp of creamed horseradish
- 85g of watercress (large stalks removed)

Steps

1. Preheat oven to 200°C/180°C fan/gas mark 6. Beetroot must be peeled and sliced into 8 wedges. Onions & butternut squash must be cut in the same proportion. In a wide roasting tin, put out the ingredients. Whisk together the vinegar & sugar until fully dissolved, then add the oil. Pour over the vegetables, toss, and roast for 40-45 minutes, stirring halfway through cooking, until charred and tender.
2. To make the horseradish cream, mix horseradish, soured cream, lemon juice, and seasonings in a mixing bowl.
3. For serving, mix the roasted vegetables with the watercress in a big bowl or on a platter, then drizzle with the horseradish cream. Hot or cold, both are fine.

5.13. Healthy Egg And Chips

Cooking time: 1 hour

Servings: 4

Difficulty level: Medium

ngredients

- 1 tbsp of olive oil
- 2 shallots (sliced)
- 2 tsp oregano (dried crushed or fresh leaves)
- 200g of small mushroom

- 4 eggs
- 500g potatoes (diced)

Steps

1. Preheat oven to 200°C/180°C fan/gas mark 6. Place the potatoes & shallots in a big non-stick roasting pan, drizzle with oil, and season with oregano, then toss well. Bake for 40-45 minutes (or when the potatoes are beginning to brown), then add the mushrooms and cook for another 10 minutes, or until the potatoes become browned and soft.
2. Cut four holes in the vegetables, then put the eggs into each. Return the eggs to the oven for another 3-4 minutes, or until they are fried to your taste.

5.14. Baked Eggs With Tomato & Spinach

Cooking time: 15 minutes

Servings: 4

Difficulty level: Easy

Ingredients

- 400g-can tomatoes (chopped)
- 4 eggs
- 100g bag spinach
- 1 tsp chili flakes

Steps

1. Preheat the oven to 200 °c/180 °c fan/gas 6. In a large non-stick roasting pan, mix the potatoes and shallots, drizzle with oil, then season with oregano, and toss well. Cook for the next 10 minutes, or when the potatoes start to brown and tender, after baking for about 40-45 minutes (or until the potatoes are starting to brown).
2. Poke four holes in the vegetables, one for each egg. Put the eggs in the oven for 3-4 minutes more, or until they are fried to your preference.

5.15. Creamy Pumpkin And Lentil Soup

Cooking time: 35 minutes

Servings: 4

Difficulty level: Easy

Ingredients

- Pinch of salt & sugar
- About 800g pumpkin flesh (chopped plus the seeds)
- 50g crème fraîche, (plus extra to serve)
- 2 onions (chopped)
- 2 garlic cloves (chopped)
- 1l of hot vegetable stock
- 100g of split red lentil
- 1 tbsp of olive oil (plus 1 tsp)
- ½ small pack thyme, (leaves picked)

Steps

1. In a large dish, heat the oil. Fry fresh onions until they are softened and golden. Pour in the hot stock after whisking in the garlic, pumpkin flesh, lentils, and thyme. Season with salt and pepper, cover, cook for 20-25 minutes, or until the lentils & vegetables become soft.
2. In the meantime, clean the pumpkin seeds. Remove any remaining flesh, then pat them dry with kitchen paper. In a non-stick skillet, heat 1 tsp oil and fry the seeds until they appear to hop and pop. Stir constantly; however, cover the pan while stirrings to keep the ingredients protected. Add a touch of sugar and a sprinkling of salt when the seeds appear nutty and toasted, and mix well.
3. Whizz the pumpkin (cooked) mixture until creamy, then apply the whizz again and crème fraîche. Season to taste.
4. Garnish with a dollop of crème fraîche, a scattering of toasted seeds and a few thyme leaves,

5.16. Asian Chicken Salad

Cooking time: 10 minutes

Servings: 2

Difficulty level: Easy

Ingredients

- Zest & juice ½ lime (about 1 tbsp)
- Large handful of coriander (roughly chopped)
- 100g bag of mixed salad leaves
- 1 tsp of caster sugar
- 1 tbsp of fish sauce
- 1 chicken breast (boneless, skinless)
- ½ chili (deseeded & thinly sliced)
- ¼ red onion
- ¼ cucumber (sliced lengthways)

Steps

1. Place the chicken in a pot of cold water, then bring to a boil and simmer for 10 minutes. Remove the meat from a pan and shred it. Stir the lime zest, fish sauce, juice, and sugar together until the sugar is dissolved.
2. In a container, mix the leaves and coriander, then cover with the chicken, pepper, onion and cucumber. Toss the salad with dressing in a different pan until preparing to serve.

5.17. Blueberry Compote With Porridge

Cooking time: 5 minutes

Servings: 2

Difficulty level: Easy

Ingredients

- 0% fat yogurt
- ½ x 350g pack frozen blueberries
- tbsp of porridge oats
- **Optional**: 1 tsp honey

Steps

1. In a non-stick pan, mix the oats in 400ml water and cook, stirring regularly, for around 2

minutes, or until thickened. Take the pan off the heat and whisk in a quarter of the yogurt.

2. In the meantime, gently poach the blueberries in a pan with 2 tsp water and the sugar, if used, until they have thawed and are soft but still retain their form.
3. Divide the Porridge among cups, cover with the remaining yogurt, and scatter the blueberries on top.

5.18. Moroccan Chickpea Soup

Cooking time: 20 minutes

Servings: 4

Difficulty level: Easy

Ingredients

- Zest & juice ½ lemon
- Large handful coriander (or parsley & flatbread for serving)
- 600ml of hot vegetable stock
- 400g can of plum tomatoes with garlic (chopped)
- 400g-can chickpeas (rinsed & drained)
- 2 tsp of ground cumin
- 2 celery sticks (chopped)
- 100g of frozen broad beans
- 1 tbsp of olive oil
- 1 onion (chopped)

Steps

1. In a big saucepan, heat the oil and gently fry the onion & celery for 10 minutes, or until softened, stirring constantly. Add the cumin and cook for another minute.
2. Increase the heat to high, and add the stock, tomatoes, and chickpeas, along with a generous pinch of black pepper. Cook for 8 minutes. Cook for another 2 minutes after adding the broad beans & lemon juice. Season with salt and pepper, then garnish with lemon zest and the chopped herbs. With flatbread, if desired.

5.19. Chunky Butternut Mulligatawny

Cooking time: 40 minutes

Servings: 6

Difficulty level: Easy

Ingredients

- Small pack parsley (chopped)
- Natural yogurt (to serve)
- 3 celery sticks (finely chopped)
- 2-3 heaped tbsp of gluten-free curry powder (depending on the extent of spiciness)
- 2 × 400g cans of chopped tomatoes
- 2 tbsp of olive or rapeseed oil
- 2 onions of finely chopped
- 2 dessert apples of peeled & finely chopped
- 140g of basmati rice
- 1 tbsp of nigella seeds (also known as a black onion or the kalonji seeds)
- 1 tbsp of ground cinnamon
- 1 ½ pound of gluten-free chicken or vegetable stock
- ½ small of butternut squash (peeled, chopped into small pieces
- Seeds removed)
- **Option**: 3 tbsp of mango chutney (plus a little to serve)

Steps

1. In the biggest saucepan, heat the oil. With a sprinkle of flour, toss in the carrots, apples, and celery. Cook and stir for 10 minutes, or until softened. Mix the butternut squash, cinnamon, nigella seeds, curry powder, and black pepper pinch in a mixing bowl. Cook for another 2 minutes, then add the tomatoes & stock. Simmer for 15 minutes with the cover on.
2. The vegetables must be soft but not mushy at this stage. Stir in the rice, cover, and continue to

3. cook for another 12 minutes or until the rice is tender. If necessary, season with more salt and pepper. Stir in the parsley & mango chutney, then serve in bowls with extra mango chutney and yogurt on top, if desired.

5.20. Spinach And Pepper Frittata

Cooking time: 40 minutes

Servings: 4

Difficulty level: Easy

Ingredients

- 5 large eggs
- 300g of low-fat cottage cheese
- 225g frozen leaf spinach (squeezed, thawed, & finely chopped)
- 2 roasted red peppers (torn into strips)
- 15g parmesan or any vegetarian alternative (finely grated)
- 100g of whole cherry tomato
- 1 garlic clove (finely chopped)
- Grating of nutmeg (generous)

Steps

1. Preheat the oven to 190°C/170°C fan/gas mark 1 5. If your sandwich tin has a loose rim, line it with a single sheet of baking parchment.
2. In a big mixing cup, whisk together the eggs, garlic, cottage cheese, half of the Parmesan, spinach,
3. nutmeg, pepper and black pepper. Fill the tray halfway with the mixture, then top with tomatoes and the leftover Parmesan. Bake about 40 minutes, or until fully set and beginning to puff up.
4. You can serve hot or cold after cutting into wedges. In the fridge, it will last 3-4 days.

5.21. Mediterranean Chunky Tomato Soup

Cooking time: 40 minutes

Servings: 4

Difficulty level: Easy

Ingredients

- 1 vegetable stock cube (reduced-salt)
- 2 tbsp of chopped garlic
- 400g of can chopped tomato
- 400g frozen grilled vegetable mix (aubergine, onion, peppers, courgettes)
- 50g of ricotta per person (basil, spread on a slice of rye bread and beaten with snipped chives)
- Handful basil leaves

Steps

1. In a large non-stick skillet, heat half of the vegetables and the garlic over high heat, constantly stirring, until they begin to soften, around 5 minutes. Add the basil, onions, stock cube, and 2 cans of water, and blitz the mixture with a hand blender until it's as smooth as possible.
2. Add the frozen vegetables, cover, and cook for another 15-20 minutes, or until the vegetables are tender. Pour into serving dishes. On rye bread, spread the herby ricotta and serve.

5.22. Griddled Vegetable And Feta Tart

Cooking time: 40 minutes

Servings: 4

Difficulty level: Easy

Ingredients

- 1 sliced aubergine
- 1 tsp of dried oregano
- 10-12 cherry tomatoes (halved)
- 2 sliced courgettes
- Two red onions (chunky wedges)
- 2 tbsp of olive oil
- 3 large sheets of filo pastry
- 85g feta cheese (crumbled)
- A drizzle of the balsamic vinegar
- Low-fat dressing and a large bag of mixed salad leaves (o serve)

Steps

1. Preheat oven to 220°C/200°C fan/gas mark 7. Preheat the oven to 350°F and place a 33 x 23cm baking tray inside. Griddle the aubergines when nicely charred in a griddle pan with around 1 tsp oil, then peel. Using a little more oil if necessary, repeat with both the courgettes and onions.
2. Take the tray out of the oven and lightly oil it. Brush a big sheet of filo with oil, layer another sheet on top, drizzle with some more oil, and repeat with a final sheet. Place the pastry on the

hot tray and gently press it into the corners.

3. Arrange the griddled vegetables on top, then season with salt and pepper. Drizzle the vinegar and any leftover oil over the tomatoes, cut-side up. Sprinkle oregano and crumbled feta on top. Cook for about 20 minutes, or until golden and crispy. Serve with the blended salad leaves that have been dressed.

5.23. Spiced Pepper Pilafs

Cooking time: 50 minutes

Servings: 8

Difficulty level: Easy

Ingredients

- 1 onion (finely chopped)
- 1 tbsp of vegetable oil
- 1 tsp of garam masala
- 1 tsp of ground cumin
- 1 tsp of tomato purée
- 140g red lentils (washed & drained)
- 1cm piece ginger (finely chopped)
- 2 garlic cloves (crushed)
- 200g bag of spinach leaves (chopped)
- 200g of basmati rice
- peppers
- 850ml vegetable stock

- Handful mint leaves (chopped)

Steps

1. In a big saucepan with a filter, heat the oil. Cook for 5 minutes until the garlic, onion, and ginger have softened. Cook for 1 minute more after adding the tomato spices and purée. Pour throughout the stock and stir to coat the rice. Bring to a boil, then add the lentils, cover and cook on low heat for 15 minutes, or until the lentils & rice are cooked. Mix the spinach with mint in a bowl and mix.
2. Remove the tops of each pepper with a sharp knife. Cut a middle stalk and any seeds with a

knife. Trim the bottom slightly so they remain upright, but not so far that the filling falls out. Fill every pepper with the rice mixture and cover with the lid. Bake or you can freeze in firmly wrapped in cling film or foil pouches.

3. If using frozen peppers, defrost entirely before cooking. Preheat oven to 200°C/180°C fan/gas mark 6. Place the peppers on a baking tray (gently oiled) and bake for 25-30 minutes or until softened. Toss a green salad with cucumber, herbs, and a spoonful of yogurt before serving.

5.24. Mustardy Beetroot & Lentil Salad

Cooking time: 20 minutes

Servings: 5 to 6

Difficulty level: Easy

Ingredients

- large handful tarragon, roughly chopped
- 300g pack cooked beetroot (not in vinegar), sliced
- 1 ½ tbsp extra virgin olive oil
- 1 tbsp wholegrain mustard (or gluten-free alternative)
- 200 g puy lentils (pre-cooked lentil 2 x 250 g packs)

Steps

1. If you're not using pre-cooked lentils, cook them according to the package directions, then drain and cool. In the meanwhile, produce a dressing with mustard, grease, and some seasoning.
2. Pour the dressing over the lentils in a mixing bowl and stir well. Serve with the beets, tarragon, and a pinch of salt and pepper.

5.25. Mushroom, Spinach & Potato Pie

Cooking time: 45 minutes

Servings: 4

Difficulty level: Easy

Ingredients

- 300g each green beans and broccoli, steamed
- 2 heaped tbsp light crème fraîche
- 3 sheets filo pastry
- 1 tbsp grain mustard
- 1 tsp freshly grated nutmeg
- 250ml vegetable stock (made from half a low sodium vegetable stock cube)
- 300g cooked new potatoes, cut into bite-sized pieces
- 500g mushroom, such as chestnut, shiitake and button
- 2 garlic cloves, crushed
- 400g baby spinach
- 1 tbsp olive oil

Steps

1. Heat oven to 200C/180C fan/gas 6. Wilt spinach in a colander by pouring a kettleful of hot water over it.
2. Heat half the oil in a large non-stick pan and fry mushrooms on high heat until golden. Add garlic and cook for 1 min, then tip in stock, mustard, nutmeg and potatoes. Bubble for a few mins until reduced. Season, then remove from the heat; add crème fraîche and spinach. Pour into a pie dish and allow to cool for a few mins.
3. Brush filo with remaining oil, quarter sheets, then loosely scrunch up and lay on top of pie filling. Bake for 20-25 mins until golden. Serve with vegetables.

5.26. Cobb Salad With Brown Derby Dressing

Cooking time: 30 minutes

Servings: 2

Difficulty level: Easy

Ingredients

- 1/2 cup blue cheese, crumbled
- 2 tbsp chives, chopped fine
- 3 hardboiled egg
- 1 avocado, sliced in half, seeded and peeled
- 1 bunch chicory lettuce
- 1/2 head romaine lettuce
- 1/2 lb smoked turkey breast
- 2 medium tomatoes, skinned and seeded
- 1/2 head iceberg lettuce
- 1/2 bunch watercress

Dressing

- 2 cloves garlic, minced very fine
- 2 tbsp olive oil
- 1/8 tsp Dijon mustard
- 1/2 tsp fresh ground black pepper
- 1 tbsp fresh lemon juice
- 2 tbsp balsamic vinegar (or red wine vinegar)
- 1/2 tsp Worcestershire sauce
- 3/4 tsp kosher salt
- 1/8 tsp sugar
- 2 tbsps water

Steps

1. Chop all the greens very, very fine (almost minced).
2. Arrange in rows in a chilled salad bowl.
3. Cut the tomatoes in half, seed, and chop very fine.
4. Fine dice the turkey, avocado, eggs and bacon.
5. Arrange all the ingredients, including the blue cheese, in rows across the lettuces.

6. Sprinkle with the chives.
7. Present at the table in this fashion, then toss with the dressing at the very last minute and serve in chilled salad bowls.
8. Serve with fresh french bread.
9. FOR THE DRESSING: Combine all the ingredients except the olive oil in a blender and blend.
10. Slowly, with the machine running, add the oil and blend well.
11. Keep refrigerated.
12. NOTE: This dish should be kept chilled and served as chilled as possible.

5.27. Mama's Supper Club Tilapia Parmesan

Cooking time: 35 minutes

Servings: 4

Difficulty level: Easy

Ingredients

- 1 dash hot pepper sauce
- 1/4 tsp dried basil
- 1/4 tsp seasoning salt
- 3 tbsps finely chopped green onions
- 3 tbsps mayonnaise
- 4 tbsp butter, room temperature
- 1/2 cup grated parmesan cheese
- 2 tbsps lemon juice
- 2 lbs tilapia fillets (orange cod, roughy or red snapper can be replaced)

Steps

1. Preheat oven to 350°F.
2. Arrange the fillets in a single layer in a buttered 13x9-inch baking tray or jellyroll tray.
3. Fillets should not be stacked.
4. Brush the top with juice.
5. In a bowl, combine butter, mayonnaise, cheese, onions and seasonings.

6. Mix with a fork.
7. Bake the fish for 10 to 20 minutes, or before it begins to flake.
8. Spread the cheese mixture on top and bake for 5 minutes or until golden brown.
9. The time it would take to roast the fish can be calculated by its thickness.
10. Keep an eye on the fish to make sure it doesn't overcook.

Note: This fish can be cooked in a broiler as well.

11. Broil for at least 3 to 4 minutes.
12. Broil for another 2 or 3 minutes, just until cheese is browned.

Conclusion

If you adjust the duration of what you eat, it is still wise to check with a licensed healthcare provider before any dietary adjustments. They will help you figure out if intermittent fasting is right for you.

This time-restricted eating style may work for some, but it may result in an unhealthy relationship with food for others. This is particularly essential for long-term fasts that may result in mineral and vitamin depletion. It's important to recognize that our bodies are extremely intellectual.

If food is limited at one meal, the body will experience increased appetite and calorie intake at the next meal and slow our metabolism to match caloric intake. While intermittent fasting has several possible health benefits, it cannot be believed that it would result in massive weight loss and avoid the onset or worsening of the disease if strictly practiced. It's a valuable tool, but it's possible that a combination of tools would be needed to achieve and sustain optimum wellbeing. Intermittent fasting helps lose weight and promotes health. However, it is not superior to conventional calorie restriction diets, scientists have found out in the largest investigation on intermittent fasting to date.

The scientists conclude that many paths are leading to a healthier weight. Everybody must find a diet plan that fits them best and then just do it. Intermittent fasting shows promise for the treatment of obesity. To date, the studies have been small and of short duration. Longer-term research is needed to understand the sustainable role IF can play in weight loss.

CPSIA information can be obtained
at www.ICGtesting.com
Printed in the USA
BVHW010335080521
606756BV00008B/1865

9 781990 387104